THE ALPHA-GAL

ALLERGY CURE BOOK

DR. RITA BROOKS

COPYRIGHT

All rights reserved. This book or any portion thereof may not be reproduced or used in any manner whatsoever without the express written permission of the publisher except for the use of brief quotations in a book review.

TABLE OF CONTENTS

OVERVIEW 7

EVERYTHING YOU NEED TO KNOW ABOUT ALLERGIES 11

    Allergies Explained 11

    Symptoms of Allergies 12

    FOR FOOD ALLERGIES 13

    FOR SEASONAL ALLERGIES 14

    FOR SEVERE ALLERGIES 14

ALLERGIES ON SKIN 16

    Causes of Allergies 18

    HOW ALLERGIES ARE DIAGNOSED .. 22

    Allergy Blood Test 23

    Skin Test 23

Preventing Symptoms 24

Complications of Allergies 26

ASTHMA AND ALLERGIES 28

ALLERGIES VS. COLD 29

ALLERGY COUGH 31

ALLERGIES AND BRONCHITIS 32

ALLERGIES AND BABIES 34

Living with Allergies 36

ALPHA-GAL SYNDROME 37

WHEN TO SEE A DOCTOR 42

Causes 43

Diagnosis 44

Tick Bites 46

The Cancer Drug Cetuximab 47

Risk Factors 48

MANAGING THE ALPHA GAL ALLERGY . 56

Nutrition Implications of Alpha-Gal Allergy 61

How Dietitians Can Help 62

Foods to Avoid 63

Everyday Food That Provides Natural Allergy Relief................................. 66

Quercetin...................................... 67

Vitamin C...................................... 68

Bromelain 69

TREATING AND PREVENTING ALPHA-GAL ALLERGY 72

Medications.................................. 72

Identifying Diet Triggers 73

Treatment.................................... 74

PREPARING FOR YOUR APPOINTMENT . 79

WHAT TO EXPECT FROM YOUR

DOCTOR 82

WHAT YOU CAN DO IN THE MEANTIME

.... 84

HOW DO YOU PREVENT AN ALPHA-GAL

ALLERGY? 87

OVERVIEW

The most common foods that cause allergic reactions in people are milk, egg, fish, wheat, shellfish, tree nuts, peanuts, and soybeans. However, there have been reports of allergic reactions to many other types of foods, including red meat. Research shows that for a red meat allergy, unlike many food allergies, the cause can be connected to an environmental factor, a tick bite.

Alpha-gal syndrome is a recently identified type of food allergy to red meat and other products made from mammals.

In the United States, the condition is most often caused by a Lone Star tick bite. The bite transmits a sugar molecule called alpha-gal into the person's body. In some people, this triggers an immune system reaction that later produces mild to severe allergic reactions to red meat, such as beef, pork or lamb, or other mammal products.

The Lone Star tick is found predominantly in the southeastern United States, and most cases of alpha-gal syndrome occur in this region. The tick can also be found in the eastern and south central United States. The condition appears to be spreading farther north and west, however, as deer carry the Lone Star tick to new parts of the United States. Alpha-gal syndrome also has been diagnosed in Europe, Australia and Asia, where other types of ticks carry alpha-gal molecules.

Researchers now believe that some people who have frequent, unexplained anaphylactic reactions — and who test negative for other food allergies — may be affected by alpha-gal syndrome. There's no treatment other than avoiding red meat and other products made from mammals. Avoiding tick bites is the key to prevention. Protect against tick bites by wearing long pants and long-sleeved shirts and using insect repellents when you're in wooded, grassy areas. Do a thorough, full-body tick check after spending time outside.

Alpha-gal syndrome is a rare allergy to a specific type of sugar found in meat — specifically beef and pork and other types of red meat. This syndrome develops in some people after a bite from a Lone Star tick. But it is still unclear why this happens. People with AGS should avoid red meat, carry an injectable form of epinephrine in the event of a reaction, and try to avoid more tick bites. Over time, the allergy may go away on its own.

EVERYTHING YOU NEED TO KNOW ABOUT ALLERGIES

Allergies Explained

An allergy is an immune system response to a foreign substance that's not typically harmful to your body. These foreign substances are called allergens. They can include certain foods, pollen, or pet dander. Your immune system's job is to keep you healthy by fighting harmful pathogens. It does this by attacking anything it thinks could put your body in danger. Depending on the allergen, this response may involve inflammation, sneezing, or a host of other symptoms.

Your immune system normally adjusts to your environment. For example, when your body encounters something like pet dander, it should realize it's harmless. In people with dander allergies, the immune system perceives it as an outside invader threatening the body and attacks it. Allergies are common. Several treatments can help you avoid your symptoms.

Symptoms of Allergies

The symptoms you experience because of allergies are the result of several factors. These include the type of allergy you have and how severe the allergy is.

If you take any medication before an anticipated allergic response, you may still experience some of these symptoms, but they may be reduced.

FOR FOOD ALLERGIES

Food allergies can trigger swelling, hives, nausea, fatigue, and more. It may take a while for a person to realize that they have a food allergy. If you have a serious reaction after a meal and you're not sure why, see a medical professional immediately. They can find the exact cause of your reaction or refer you to a specialist.

FOR SEASONAL ALLERGIES

Hay fever symptoms can mimic those of a cold. They include congestion, runny nose, and swollen eyes. Most of the time, you can manage these symptoms at home using over-the-counter treatments. See your doctor if your symptoms become unmanageable.

FOR SEVERE ALLERGIES

Severe allergies can cause anaphylaxis. This is a life-threatening emergency that can lead to breathing difficulties, lightheadedness, and loss of consciousness. If you're experiencing these symptoms after coming in contact with a possible allergen, seek medical help immediately.

Everyone's signs and symptoms of an allergic reaction are different. Read more about allergy symptoms and what might cause them.

ALLERGIES ON SKIN

Skin allergies may be a sign or symptom of an allergy. They may also be the direct result of exposure to an allergen.

For example, eating a food you're allergic to can cause several symptoms. You may experience tingling in your mouth and throat. You may also develop a rash.

Contact dermatitis, however, is the result of your skin coming into direct contact with an allergen. This could happen if you touch something you're allergic to, such as a cleaning product or plant.

Types of skin allergies include:

Rashes. Areas of skin are irritated, red, or swollen, and can be painful or itchy.

Eczema. Patches of skin become inflamed and can itch and bleed.

Contact dermatitis. Red, itchy patches of skin develop almost immediately after contact with an allergen.

Sore throat. Pharynx or throat is irritated or inflamed.

Hives. Red, itchy, and raised welts of various sizes and shapes develop on the surface of the skin.

Swollen eyes. Eyes may be watery or itchy and look "puffy."

Itching. There's irritation or inflammation in the skin.

Burning. Skin inflammation leads to discomfort and stinging sensations on the skin.

Rashes are one of the most common symptoms of a skin allergy. Find out how to identify rashes and how to treat them.

Causes of Allergies

Researchers aren't exactly sure why the immune system causes an allergic reaction when a normally harmless foreign substance enters the body.

Allergies have a genetic component. This means parents can pass them down to their children. However, only a general susceptibility to allergic reaction is genetic. Specific allergies aren't passed down. For instance, if your mother is allergic to shellfish, it doesn't necessarily mean that you'll be, too.

Common types of allergens include:

- Animal products. These include pet dander, dust mite waste, and cockroaches.

- Drugs. Penicillin and sulfa drugs are common triggers.

- Foods. Wheat, nuts, milk, shellfish, and egg allergies are common.

- Insect stings. These include bees, wasps, and mosquitoes.

- Mold. Airborne spores from mold can trigger a reaction.

- Plants. Pollens from grass, weeds, and trees, as well as resin from plants such as poison ivy and poison oak, are very common plant allergens.

- Other allergens. Latex, often found in latex gloves and condoms, and metals like nickel are also common allergens.

Seasonal allergies, also known as hay fever, are some of the most common allergies. These are caused by pollen released by plants. They cause:

- itchy eyes

- watery eyes

- runny nose

- coughing

Food allergies are becoming more common. Find out about the most common types of food allergies and the symptoms they cause.

HOW ALLERGIES ARE DIAGNOSED

Your doctor can diagnose allergies in several ways.

First, your doctor will ask about your symptoms and perform a physical exam. They'll ask about anything unusual you may have eaten recently and any substances you may have come in contact with. For example, if you have a rash on your hands, your doctor may ask if you put on latex gloves recently.

Lastly, a blood test and skin test can confirm or diagnose allergens your doctor suspects you have.

Allergy Blood Test

Your doctor may order a blood test. Your blood will be tested for the presence of allergy-causing antibodies called immunoglobulin E (IgE). These are cells that react to allergens. Your doctor will use a blood test to confirm a diagnosis if they're worried about the potential for a severe allergic reaction.

Skin Test

Your doctor may also refer you to an allergist for testing and treatment. A skin test is a common type of allergy test carried out by an allergist.

During this test, your skin is pricked or scratched with small needles containing potential allergens. Your skin's reaction is documented. If you're allergic to a particular substance, your skin will become red and inflamed.

Different tests may be needed to diagnose all your potential allergies. Start here to get a better understanding of how allergy testing works.

Preventing Symptoms

There's no way to prevent allergies. But there are ways to prevent the symptoms from occurring. The best way to prevent allergy symptoms is to avoid the allergens that trigger them.

Avoidance is the most effective way to prevent food allergy symptoms. An elimination diet can help you determine the cause of your allergies so you know how to avoid them. To help you avoid food allergens, thoroughly read food labels and ask questions while dining out.

Preventing seasonal, contact, and other allergies comes down to knowing where the allergens are located and how to avoid them. If you're allergic to dust, for example, you can help reduce symptoms by installing proper air filters in your home, getting your air ducts professionally cleaned, and dusting your home regularly.

Proper allergy testing can help you pinpoint your exact triggers, which makes them easier to avoid. These other tips can also help you avoid dangerous allergic reactions.

Complications of Allergies

While you may think of allergies as those pesky sniffles and sneezes that come around every new season, some of these allergic reactions can actually be life-threatening.

Anaphylaxis, for example, is a serious reaction to the exposure of allergens. Most people associate anaphylaxis with food, but any allergen can cause the telltale signs:

- suddenly narrowed airways

- increased heart rate

- possible swelling of the tongue and mouth

Allergy symptoms can create many complications. Your doctor can help determine the cause of your symptoms as well as the difference between a sensitivity and a full-blown allergy. Your doctor can also teach you how to manage your allergy symptoms so that you can avoid the worst complications.

ASTHMA AND ALLERGIES

Asthma is a common respiratory condition. It makes breathing more difficult and can narrow the air passageways in your lungs.

Asthma is closely related to allergies. Indeed, allergies can make existing asthma worse. It can also trigger asthma in a person who's never had the condition.

When these conditions occur together, it's a condition called allergy-induced asthma, or allergic asthma. Allergic asthma affects about 60 percent of people who have asthma in the United States, estimates the Allergy and Asthma Foundation of America.

Many people with allergies may develop asthma. Here's how to recognize if it happens to you.

ALLERGIES VS. COLD

Runny nose, sneezing, and coughing are common symptoms of allergies. They also happen to be common symptoms of a cold and a sinus infection. Indeed, deciphering between the sometimes-generic symptoms can be difficult.

However, additional signs and symptoms of the conditions may help you distinguish between the three. For example, allergies can cause rashes on your skin and itchy eyes. The common cold can lead to body aches, even fever. A sinus infection typically produces thick, yellow discharge from your nose.

Allergies can impact your immune system for prolonged periods of time. When the immune system is compromised, it makes you more likely to pick up viruses you come into contact with. This includes the virus that causes the common cold.

In turn, having allergies actually increases your risk for having more colds. Identify the differences between the two common conditions with this helpful chart.

ALLERGY COUGH

Hay fever can produce symptoms that include sneezing, coughing, and a persistent, stubborn cough. It's the result of your body's overreaction to allergens. It isn't contagious, but it can be miserable. Unlike a chronic cough, a cough caused by allergies and hay fever is temporary. You may only experience the symptoms of this seasonal allergy during specific times of the year, when plants are first blooming.

Additionally, seasonal allergies can trigger asthma, and asthma can cause coughing. When a person with common seasonal allergies is exposed to an allergen, tightening airways can lead to a cough. Shortness of breath and chest tightening may also occur.

Find out why hay fever coughs are typically worse at night and what you can do to ease them.

ALLERGIES AND BRONCHITIS

Viruses or bacteria can cause bronchitis, or it can be the result of allergies. The first type, acute bronchitis, typically ends after several days or weeks. Chronic bronchitis, however, can linger for months, possibly longer. It may also return frequently.

Exposure to common allergens is the most common cause of chronic bronchitis. These allergens include:

- cigarette smoke

- air pollution

- dust

- pollen

- chemical fumes

Unlike seasonal allergies, many of these allergens linger in environments like houses or offices. That can make chronic bronchitis more persistent and more likely to return.

A cough is the only common symptom between chronic and acute bronchitis. Learn the other symptoms of bronchitis so you can understand more clearly what you may have.

ALLERGIES AND BABIES

Skin allergies are more common in younger children today than they were just a few decades ago. However, skin allergies decrease as children grow older. Respiratory and food allergies become more common as children get older.

Common skin allergies on babies include:

Eczema. This is an inflammatory skin condition that causes red rashes that itch. These rashes may develop slowly but be persistent.

Allergic contact dermatitis. This type of skin allergy appears quickly, often immediately after your baby comes into contact with the irritant. More serious contact dermatitis can develop into painful blisters and cause skin cracking.

Hives. Hives are red bumps or raised areas of skin that develop after exposure to an allergen. They don't become scaly and crack, but itching the hives may make the skin bleed.

Unusual rashes or hives on your baby's body may alarm you. Understanding the difference in the type of skin allergies babies commonly experience can help you find a better treatment.

Living with Allergies

Allergies are common and don't have life-threatening consequences for most people. People who are at risk of anaphylaxis can learn how to manage their allergies and what to do in an emergency situation. Most allergies are manageable with avoidance, medications, and lifestyle changes. Working with your doctor or allergist can help reduce any major complications and make life more enjoyable.

ALPHA-GAL SYNDROME

Alpha-gal syndrome is an allergy to things like beef, pork, lamb, venison, rabbit, and other animal products that come from mammals. It was first discovered in 2009. Alpha galactose, the source of the allergy, is a sugar present in most animal cells. Alpha-gal symptoms develop after certain tick bites. The best way to diagnose alpha-gal allergy is with a blood test measuring alpha-gal antibodies. Other pertinent history includes recent outdoor activity, exposure to ticks, and any known or suspected reaction after consuming mammalian meats.

Alpha-gal allergic reaction symptoms are similar to those of any food allergy with one notable exception: alpha-gal reaction symptoms can be delayed by two to six hours after exposure to mammalian meats. If symptoms are delayed, it can confuse patients, family members, and clinicians when attempting to track the cause of the allergic reaction. The most common symptom reported is typically skin reactions, but reactions can be as severe as anaphylaxis. Adults appear to have more severe reactions than children do.

Symptoms

Signs and symptoms of an alpha-gal allergic reaction are often delayed compared with other food allergies. Most reactions to common food allergens — peanuts or shellfish, for example — happen within minutes of exposure. In alpha-gal syndrome, reactions usually appear about three to six hours after exposure. Red meat, such as beef, pork or lamb; organ meats; and products made from mammals, such as gelatins or dairy products, can cause a reaction.

Signs and symptoms of alpha-gal syndrome may include:

- Hives, itching, or itchy, scaly skin (eczema)

- Swelling of the lips, face, tongue and throat, or other body parts

- Wheezing or shortness of breath

- A runny nose

- Stomach pain, diarrhea, nausea or vomiting

- Sneezing

- Headaches

- A severe, potentially deadly allergic reaction that restricts breathing(anaphylaxis)

Doctors think the time delay between eating red meat and developing an allergic reaction is one reason the condition was overlooked until recently. A possible connection between a T-bone steak with dinner and hives at midnight was far from obvious.

WHEN TO SEE A DOCTOR

See your primary care doctor or a doctor who specializes in the diagnosis and treatment of allergies (allergist) if you experience food allergy symptoms after eating — even several hours after eating. Don't rule out red meat as a possible cause of your reaction, especially if you live or spend time outdoors in the southeastern United States or in other parts of the world where alpha-gal syndrome is known to occur.

Seek emergency medical treatment if you develop signs or symptoms of anaphylaxis, such as:

- Difficulty breathing

- Rapid, weak pulse

- Dizziness or lightheadedness

- Drooling and inability to swallow

- Full-body redness and warmth (flushing)

Causes

A Lone Star tick bite most commonly causes the condition in the U.S. Bites from other types of ticks can lead to the condition in the U.S., Europe, Australia and Asia.

Diagnosis

Doctors can diagnose alpha-gal syndrome using a combination of your personal history and certain medical tests. Your doctor will likely start by asking about your exposure to ticks, your signs and symptoms, and how long it took for symptoms to develop after you ate red meat or other mammal products. He or she might also perform a physical exam.

Additional tests used in the evaluation of alpha-gal syndrome may include:

Blood test. A blood test can confirm and measure the amount of alpha-gal antibodies in your bloodstream. This is the key test for diagnosis of alpha-gal syndrome.

Skin test. Doctors prick your skin and expose it to small amounts of substances extracted from commercial or fresh red meat. If you're allergic, you develop a raised bump (hive) at the test site on your skin. Your doctor or allergist may also test your skin for an allergic reaction to individual types of red meat because there are different kinds of allergies to meat.

Tick Bites

Ticks that cause alpha-gal syndrome are believed to carry alpha-gal molecules from the blood of the animals they commonly bite, such as cows and sheep. When a carrier tick bites a human, the tick injects alpha-gal into the person's body. For unknown reasons, some people have such a strong immune response to these molecules that they can no longer eat red meat or products made from mammals without a mild to severe allergic reaction.

People who are exposed to many tick bites over time may develop more-severe symptoms.

The Cancer Drug Cetuximab

People with antibodies related to alpha-gal syndrome can have allergic reactions to the cancer drug cetuximab (Erbitux). Cetuximab-induced cases of this condition are most common in regions with a high population of Lone Star ticks, suggesting a possible link between Lone Star tick bites and an increased vulnerability to alpha-gal syndrome. More research is needed to understand the connection between ticks that carry alpha-gal in certain regions and cases of alpha-gal syndrome that don't seem directly linked to tick bites.

Researchers think the hallmark time-delayed reaction of alpha-gal syndrome is due to the alpha-gal molecules taking longer than other allergens to be digested and enter your circulatory system.

Risk Factors

Doctors don't yet know why some people develop alpha-gal syndrome after exposure and others don't. The condition mostly occurs in the southeastern United States and parts of New York, New Jersey and New England. You're at increased risk if you live or spend time in these regions and:

- Spend a lot of time outdoors

- Have received multiple Lone Star tick bites

- Have a mast cell abnormality such as indolent systemic mastocytosis

In the past 20 to 30 years, the Lone Star tick has been found in large numbers as far north as Maine and as far west as central Texas and Oklahoma in the United States.

Alpha-gal syndrome can also occur in other parts of the world such as Europe, Australia and parts of Asia, where bites from certain types of ticks also appear to increase your risk of the condition.

Complications

Alpha-gal syndrome can cause food-induced anaphylaxis, a medical emergency that requires treatment with an epinephrine (adrenaline) injector (EpiPen, Auvi-Q, others) and a visit to the emergency room.

Anaphylaxis signs and symptoms can include:

- Constriction of airways

- Swelling of the throat that makes it difficult to breathe

- A severe drop in blood pressure (shock)

- Rapid pulse

- Dizziness, lightheadedness or loss of consciousness

Based on recent research, doctors now believe that some people with unexplained, frequent anaphylaxis may be living with undiagnosed alpha-gal syndrome.

Precautions

The best way to prevent alpha-gal syndrome is to avoid areas where ticks live, especially wooded, bushy areas with long grass. You can decrease your risk of getting alpha-gal syndrome with some simple precautions:

Cover up. When in wooded or grassy areas, wear shoes, long pants tucked into your socks, a long-sleeved shirt, a hat and gloves. Try to stick to trails and avoid walking through low bushes and long grass. Keep your dog on a leash.

Use insect repellents. Apply insect repellent with a 20% or higher concentration of DEET to your skin. Parents should apply repellent to their children, avoiding their hands, eyes and mouths. Keep in mind that chemical repellents can be toxic, so follow directions carefully. Apply products with permethrin to clothing or buy pre-treated clothing.

Do your best to tick-proof your yard. Clear brush and leaves where ticks live. Keep woodpiles in sunny areas.

Check yourself, your children and your pets for ticks. Be especially vigilant after spending time in wooded or grassy areas. It's helpful to shower as soon as you come indoors. Ticks often remain on your skin for hours before attaching themselves. Showering and using a washcloth might remove unattached ticks.

Remove a tick as soon as possible with tweezers. Gently grasp the tick near its head or mouth. Don't squeeze or crush the tick, but pull carefully and steadily. Once you've removed the entire tick, dispose of it and apply antiseptic to the bite area.

Alpha-gal syndrome doesn't go away, but you can manage symptoms by avoiding:

• Meats, organs, and blood of mammals

• Dairy products

• Gelatin and other animal derivatives

• Food cooked with lard

• Any food with any sort of mammalian product

- Drugs, medicines, hygiene products, and household products with animal bi-products

- Anything with the thickening agent carrageenan

- Flounder eggs

You can take antihistamines or another type of allergy medicine to manage your symptoms if you have a reaction. However, if you are having an extremely severe reaction, you will need to be injected with epinephrine or even go to the emergency room. Many people with alpha-gal even carry around an EpiPen.

MANAGING THE ALPHA GAL ALLERGY

Ticks are a pest control nightmare. Not only do they carry diseases such as Lyme Disease and Rocky Mountain Spotted Fever but they are also thought to be the root cause of Multiple Sclerosis. There are dozens of species living throughout the United States and scientists have now discovered yet another reason to fear ticks. Bites from the Lone Star tick can cause an allergy to red meat.

According to researchers in Nashville at a prestigious Asthma and Allergy Clinic at Vanderbilt University, there are several cases each week reported of sudden onset of allergic reactions to red meat caused by tick bites. Imagine you're a happy beef eater and after receiving a tick bite you now cannot tolerate red meat. How does this happen?

Alpha-Galactose, commonly referred to as alpha-gal is a sugar contained in red meat. If there is an allergy to alpha-gal, a victim's body will create alpha-gal antibodies and these numbers can soar up to 20 times normal antibody levels. The allergic reaction to this sugar occurs between 4 - 8 hours after eating red meat. Reactions vary from patient to patient and can range from diarrhea and nausea/vomiting all the way through hives and difficulty breathing. Severe reactions include anaphylactic shock and even death. This is not something to take lightly!

When the allergy to this sugar is activated, the antibody count to this sugar can soar up to 20 times the normal level. The severity of reactions is in direct proportion to the spike in antibody count. What are the details on Lone Star ticks? They live throughout the southeastern United States and have been found from Texas to Maine.

Their numbers have steadily grown throughout the last 20 - 30 years along with increases in other tick species. Like other ticks, they prefer wooded areas dotted with large trees and dense under growth. The females have a distinct white star on their back which differs from other tick species. If there is any consolation in this situation, it is that the Lone Star Tick is not a known carrier of Lyme Disease.

To avoid bites from the Lone Star tick, it is advised that long sleeves and pants legs be worn when venturing into wooded areas. After exiting a forested area, do a detailed search on your entire body for ticks. They will feed on humans and domestic animals in all life stages of larva, nymph and adult and can be very aggressive feeders.

So what is the solution? Safe, green and eco-friendly tick repellents. Many websites list DEET or permethrin based products but these synthetic solutions are not safe and have been losing effectiveness. It is best to use proven, natural products which you should apply liberally and frequently if exposed to tick habitats.

Nutrition Implications of Alpha-Gal Allergy

When it comes right down to it, alpha-gal allergy is a food allergy. In theory, the treatment of alpha-gal allergy is simple—avoid offending foods. In practice, however, this can present a challenge. Once alpha-gal allergy is diagnosed, all mammalian meats and by-products should be avoided. Again, this includes, beef, pork, lamb, venison, mutton, goat, and bison, plus any food that contains red meat extracts. Some individuals with alpha-gal allergy must also avoid dairy products made from cow's, sheep's or goat's milk. The good news is that all fruits, vegetables, grains, nuts, legumes, poultry, and seafood are appropriate for alpha-gal allergies.

How Dietitians Can Help

Just like any food allergy, the long list of "no" foods can be daunting and discouraging for patients and their families. Dietitians should be equipped with an even longer list of "yes" foods that are appropriate for an alpha-gal allergy. Encourage all family members to support their loved one as they cope with their new diet restrictions. Teach clients and families how to read food labels, especially for "unsuspecting" foods like gelatin, broths, and gravies.

Make sure your client's diet is still nutritionally complete, recommending vitamin or mineral supplements, if needed. And educate the foodservice team that a red meat allergy is, indeed, a thing and what alternative food options they can safely offer.

Foods to Avoid

Knowing what to avoid after an alpha gal diagnosis is key to living you best life. Here is a basic list of foods to avoid:

- Beef

- Beef stock or broth (caution with chicken broth; ("natural flavoring" can be mammal sourced)

- Bison

- Buffalo

- Brown gravy (made with beef broth)

- Gelatin-when made from byproducts of meat and leather industry

- Certain vaccines

- Gummy Candies (unless VEGAN)

- Some ice cream and yogurt

- Gelatin Desserts

- Marshmallows

- Altoids brand mints

- Gelatin Capsules (vitamins, supplements, and RX meds in gelatin capsules)

- Medications that contain pre-gelatinized starch

- Goat

- Lamb

- Lard (some refried beans contain lard)

- Pork

- Venison

Avoid contact in a few extreme cases:

- Lanolin (sheep)

- Leather (shoes, couches, coats)

- pets/animal contact/inhalation can trigger cough

ALLOWED:

- Chicken
- Turkey
- Other birds
- Fish

Everyday Food That Provides Natural Allergy Relief

We all know that a healthy diet can do wonders for your body. Eating the right food makes your skin look better, it reduces the risk of several illnesses and it makes your body function better in general. But did you know that eating the right food can also aid you with seasonal allergies.

Though food isn't a proven cure for allergies, the nutrients they contain can help your body run at a healthy pace.

For natural edible allergy relief, try these:

Quercetin

Quercetin is an antioxidant-rich chemical that's found in natural plants. It's tied to managing aging and inflammation. Research has shown that foods containing quercetin can assist with many inflammatory issues, including allergies, asthma and hay fever. It's a natural antihistamine so it helps fight the histamine that's released when your immune system detects an allergy – which is why it's so effective for lowering allergic reactions.

Foods that contain Quercetin: Raw red Onions, Peppers, Berries, Parsley, Apples, Tomatoes, Citrus Fruits, Spinach, and Kale.

Vitamin C

Like Quercetin, Vitamin C is a natural antihistamine that is present in certain foods. The vitamin is often used to prevent and treat several illnesses: this includes allergies. It does this by lowering histamine levels in the bloodstream which prevent symptoms.

Foods that contain Vitamin C: Kiwi, Oranges and other citrus fruit

Bromelain

Bromelain is a mixture of enzymes that digest protein. Bromelain can be used to treat indigestion and reduce inflammation. For allergy sufferers, it can reduce irritation in allergic symptoms such as asthma.

Food that contain Vitamin C: Pineapple

Omega 3

There are many fatty things out there that you may want to reduce, Omega-3 fatty shouldn't be included in those. These fatty acids have several health benefits related to anti-inflammatory properties.

Foods that contain Omega-3 fatty acids: Tuna, Salmon, and mackerel

Local Honey

There's research that shows that local honey helps seasonal allergies. Taking small doses of local honey early in the season may build your tolerance toward the pollen in your area.

As stated before, these foods aren't a proven cure, but they are worth a try.

TREATING AND PREVENTING ALPHA-GAL ALLERGY

Medications

Allergic reactions to alpha-gal can be treated with an over-the-counter antihistamine such as diphenhydramine (Benadryl). Stronger reactions provoked by alpha-gal might need to be addressed with epinephrine.

Researchers don't know yet how long after the tick bite the allergy can last. Right now, they don't believe that it's chronic. However, they do point out that additional tick bites can bring the allergy back even if it becomes inactive.

Identifying Diet Triggers

If you find out that you have an alpha-gal allergy, get to work identifying your triggers. While all sorts of red meat might need to stay off your table for the time being, there could be other trigger foods that will provoke your symptoms. Dairy products, for example, can contain alpha-gal.

People with any serious food allergy should be hyperaware of what's in their food. If your symptoms are serious when you have an allergic reaction, you might want to start carrying a portable epinephrine treatment (such as an EpiPen) in case of an emergency. Make sure that your family, co-workers, and people you live with know what to do if you have a severe allergic reaction. Go over possible action plans with them before you need their help.

Treatment

Immediate symptoms such as hives or shortness of breath are treated the same as any other food allergy - in an urgent care setting with anti-histamines, epinephrine and other medications. Prevention long-term involves avoidance of all red meat in sensitized individuals. You may be advised to carry an epinephrine auto-injector, to be used in case of subsequent accidental exposures and reaction. These measures do not necessarily mean switching to a full vegetarian diet, since poultry and fish can be consumed and do not cause similar reactions. As with other food allergies, there is the possibility that over time the sensitivity diminishes – although these changes may take many years to become apparent.

As with any food allergy, alpha-gal syndrome treatment involves avoiding the foods that cause your reaction. Always check the ingredient labels on store-bought foods to make sure they don't contain red meat or meat-based ingredients, such as beef, pork, lamb, organ meats or gelatins.

Check soup stock cubes, gravy packages and flavor ingredients in prepackaged products. Ask your doctor or allergist for a list of foods to avoid, including meat extracts used in flavoring. The names of some ingredients make them difficult to recognize as meat based.

Use extra caution when you eat at restaurants and social gatherings. Many people don't understand the seriousness of an allergic food reaction, and few realize meat allergies even exist.

Even a small amount of red meat can cause a severe reaction.

If you are at all worried that a food may contain something you're allergic to, don't try it. Come prepared to social events to avoid risk of exposure. For example, if you're attending a party where guests prepare food on a shared cooking surface, bring your own precooked food.

For a severe allergic reaction, you may need an emergency injection of epinephrine and a visit to the emergency room. Many people with allergies carry an epinephrine autoinjector (EpiPen,

Auvi-Q, others). This device is a syringe and concealed needle that injects a single dose of medication when pressed against the thigh. Once you've been diagnosed with alpha-gal syndrome, your doctor or allergist likely will prescribe an epinephrine autoinjector.

Symptoms of alpha-gal syndrome may lessen or even disappear over time if you don't get any more bites from ticks that carry alpha-gal. Some people with this condition have been able to eat red meat and other mammal products again after one to two years without additional bites.

PREPARING FOR YOUR APPOINTMENT

To get the most from your appointment, it's a good idea to be well prepared. Here's some information to help you get ready for your appointment and to know what to expect from your doctor.

Description of your symptoms. Be ready to tell your doctor what happened after you ate red meat, including how long it took for a reaction to occur. Be prepared to describe the type of red meat you ate as well as the portion size.

History of tick bites or possible exposure to ticks. Your doctor will need to know where you've spent time outdoors and how often, as well as how many tick bites you're aware of having experienced.

Make a list of all medications you're taking. Include vitamins or supplements.

Take a family member or friend along, if possible. Sometimes it can be difficult to recall all the information provided to you during an appointment. Someone who comes with you may remember something you missed or forgot.

Write down any questions you have.

Some basic questions to ask your doctor include:

- Are my symptoms likely caused by a red meat allergy?

- What else might be causing my symptoms?

- What tests do I need?

- What's the best treatment?

- Should I see a specialist?

- Is there a generic alternative to the medicine you're prescribing?

- Are there brochures or other printed material that I can take with me? What websites do you recommend?

- Do I need to carry an epinephrine autoinjector?

WHAT TO EXPECT FROM YOUR DOCTOR

Your doctor is likely to ask you a number of questions, including:

• When did you begin noticing symptoms?

• What type of meat and how much did you eat before symptoms appeared?

• After eating red meat, how long did it take symptoms to appear?

• Are you currently spending time or have you in the past spent time outdoors in tick-infested areas?

- Have you been bitten by a tick in the past? How many times? What did these ticks look like?

- Did you take any over-the-counter allergy medications, such as antihistamines, and if so, did they help?

- Does your reaction seem to be triggered only by red meat or by other foods as well?

- How severe are your symptoms?

- What, if anything, seems to improve your symptoms?

- What, if anything, appears to worsen your symptoms?

WHAT YOU CAN DO IN THE MEANTIME

If you suspect you have alpha-gal syndrome, avoid eating red meat until your doctor's appointment. If you have a severe reaction, seek emergency help.

How do you become allergic to alpha-gal?

Alpha-gal is a molecule carried in the saliva of the Lone Star tick and other potential arthropods typically after feeding on mammalian blood. People that are bitten by the tick, especially those that are bitten repeatedly, are at risk of becoming sensitized and producing the IgE necessary to then cause allergic reactions. Interestingly, allergic reactions may occur to red meat, to subsequent tick bites, and even to medications that contain alpha-gal. Cetuximab is a cancer medication that contains alpha-gal, and people who have had allergic reactions to this medication (these are typically immediate reactions, because it is infused intravenously) have a higher risk for red meat allergy and are likely to have been bitten by ticks in the past. As might be expected, the incidence of tick bites is much higher in the southern and eastern U.S., the traditional habitat for the tick.

However, cases are now increasingly reported in the northern and western states. And it is a phenomenon that has been observed worldwide, with different ticks responsible for similar cases of red meat allergy in many other countries such as Sweden, South Africa and Australia.

The discovery of this peculiar allergy has allowed researchers to correlate tick bites with many cases of anaphylaxis that would previously have been classified as 'idiopathic', or of unknown cause. Also, while it was originally thought that the Lone Star tick had to feast on mammalian blood in order to carry the alpha-gal molecule, more recent research has shown that it may carry this molecule and be capable of sensitizing humans independently.

HOW DO YOU PREVENT AN ALPHA-GAL ALLERGY?

Because this allergy is predominantly tick born, you are more likely at risk if you often go outdoors in wooded areas for activities such as hiking, fishing or hunting. The key strategy is to prevent tick bites. This may include wearing long sleeved shirts or pants, using appropriate insect repellants, and surveying for ticks after spending time outdoors.

Any observed ticks should be removed carefully by cleaning the site with rubbing alcohol, then using tweezers to pull the tick's head up carefully from the skin using steady pressure. Clean your hands and the site one more time and make sure not to crush the tick between your fingers.

Made in United States
Orlando, FL
21 December 2024